VETERINARY CONTROLLED ~~DRUGS~~ LOG BOOK

PERSONAL DETAILS

Name : _____

Address : _____

_____

_____

Email : _____

Phone Number : _____

Fax : _____

Emergency No: _____

LOG BOOK INFORMATION

LOG BOOK START DATE	
LOG BOOK END DATE	
LOG BOOK NUMBER	

We hope that this Book will be useful and, practical as we wanted to be.

If you think that this Book is good enough, and if it had been useful in any way, please make sure to LEAVE A REVIEW ON AMAZON REVIEW SECTION.

We would definitely love to read your honest opinions, and feedback, it will make us create better products for you in the future

THANK YOU VERY MUCH FOR YOU SUPPORT.

Veterinary Controlled Substance Log

CONTROLLED SUBSTANCE : .... STRENGTH : .... FORM : ....

Date	Client, Patient	Address / ID / Serial #	Unique Botte #	Reason Notes	Admin / Dispensed By	Amount of / Waste / Hub Loss	Amount Added	Amount Used	Ending Balance
					☐ Beginning Balance Or	☐ Balance From Previous Page ⬆			

VETERINARY CONTROLLED SUBSTANCE LOG

CONTROLLED SUBSTANCE : .... STRENGTH : .... FORM : ....

Date	Client, Patient	Address / ID / Serial #	Unique Botte #	Reason Notes	Admin / Dispensed By	Amount of / Waste / Hub Loss	Amount Added	Amount Used	Ending Balance
					☐ Beginning Balance Or ☐ Balance From Previous Page ⬆				

VETERINARY CONTROLLED SUBSTANCE LOG

CONTROLLED SUBSTANCE : ....   STRENGTH : ....   FORM : ....

Date	Client, Patient Address / ID / Serial #	Unique Botte #	Reason Notes	Admin / Dispensed By	Amount of / Waste / Hub Loss	Amount Added	Amount Used	Ending Balance
				☐ Beginning Balance Or ☐ Balance From Previous Page ⇧				

VETERINARY CONTROLLED SUBSTANCE LOG

CONTROLLED SUBSTANCE : .... STRENGTH : .... FORM : ....

Date	Client, Patient	Address / ID / Serial #	Unique Botte #	Reason Notes	Admin / Dispensed By	Amount of / Waste / Hub Loss	Amount Added	Amount Used	Ending Balance
				☐ Beginning Balance Or ☐ Balance From Previous Page ⬆					

VETERINARY CONTROLLED SUBSTANCE LOG

CONTROLLED SUBSTANCE : ....   STRENGTH : ....   FORM : ....

Date	Client, Patient	Address / ID / Serial #	Unique Botte #	Reason Notes	Admin / Dispensed By	Amount of / Waste / Hub Loss	Amount Added	Amount Used	Ending Balance
					☐ Beginning Balance Or ☐ Balance From Previous Page			⇦	

VETERINARY CONTROLLED SUBSTANCE LOG

CONTROLLED SUBSTANCE : .... STRENGTH : .... FORM : ....

Date	Client, Patient	Address / ID / Serial #	Unique Botte #	Reason Notes	Admin / Dispensed By	Amount of / Waste / Hub Loss	Amount Added	Amount Used	Ending Balance
					☐ Beginning Balance Or ☐ Balance From Previous Page ⬆				

VETERINARY CONTROLLED SUBSTANCE LOG

CONTROLLED SUBSTANCE : ....   STRENGTH : ....   FORM : ....

Date	Client, Patient	Address / ID / Serial #	Unique Botte #	Reason Notes	Admin / Dispensed By	Amount of / Waste / Hub Loss	Amount Added	Amount Used	Ending Balance
					☐ Beginning Balance Or ☐ Balance From Previous Page ⇧				

Veterinary Controlled Substance Log

CONTROLLED SUBSTANCE : ....   STRENGTH : ....   FORM : ....

Date	Client, Patient	Address / ID / Serial #	Unique Botte #	Reason Notes	Admin / Dispensed By	Amount of / Waste / Hub Loss	Amount Added	Amount Used	Ending Balance
					☐ Beginning Balance Or ☐ Balance From Previous Page ⬆				

VETERINARY CONTROLLED SUBSTANCE LOG

CONTROLLED SUBSTANCE : .... STRENGTH : .... FORM : ....

Date	Client, Patient	Address / ID / Serial #	Unique Botte #	Reason Notes	Admin / Dispensed By	Amount of / Waste / Hub Loss	Amount Added	Amount Used	Ending Balance
					☐ Beginning Balance Or ☐ Balance From Previous Page			⬆	

VETERINARY CONTROLLED SUBSTANCE LOG

CONTROLLED SUBSTANCE : .... STRENGTH : .... FORM : ....

Date	Client, Patient	Address / ID / Serial #	Unique Botte #	Reason Notes	Admin / Dispensed By	Amount of / Waste / Hub Loss	Amount Added	Amount Used	Ending Balance
					☐ Beginning Balance Or ☐ Balance From Previous Page				

VETERINARY CONTROLLED SUBSTANCE LOG

CONTROLLED SUBSTANCE : .... STRENGTH : .... FORM : ....

Date	Client, Patient Address / ID / Serial #	Unique Botte #	Reason Notes	Admin / Dispensed By	Amount of / Waste / Hub Loss	Amount Added	Amount Used	Ending Balance
				☐ Beginning Balance Or ☐ Balance From Previous Page ⇦				

VETERINARY CONTROLLED SUBSTANCE LOG

CONTROLLED SUBSTANCE : .... STRENGTH : .... FORM : ....

Date	Client, Patient	Address / ID / Serial #	Unique Botte #	Reason Notes	Admin / Dispensed By	Amount of / Waste / Hub Loss	Amount Added	Amount Used	Ending Balance
					☐ Beginning Balance Or ☐ Balance From Previous Page ⇧				

VETERINARY CONTROLLED SUBSTANCE LOG

CONTROLLED SUBSTANCE : ....   STRENGTH : ....   FORM : ....

Date	Client, Patient	Address / ID / Serial #	Unique Botte #	Reason Notes	Admin / Dispensed By	Amount of / Waste / Hub Loss	Amount Added	Amount Used	Ending Balance
				☐ Beginning Balance Or	☐ Balance From Previous Page			⬆	

VETERINARY CONTROLLED SUBSTANCE LOG

CONTROLLED SUBSTANCE : ....   STRENGTH : ....   FORM : ....

Date	Client, Patient	Address / ID / Serial #	Unique Botte #	Reason Notes	Admin / Dispensed By	Amount of / Waste / Hub Loss	Amount Added	Amount Used	Ending Balance
					☐ Beginning Balance Or	☐ Balance From Previous Page			

VETERINARY CONTROLLED SUBSTANCE LOG

CONTROLLED SUBSTANCE : .... STRENGTH : .... FORM : ....

Date	Client, Patient	Address / ID / Serial #	Unique Botte #	Reason Notes	Admin / Dispensed By	Amount of / Waste / Hub Loss	Amount Added	Amount Used	Ending Balance
					☐ Beginning Balance Or ☐ Balance From Previous Page ⇧				

VETERINARY CONTROLLED SUBSTANCE LOG

CONTROLLED SUBSTANCE : .... STRENGTH : .... FORM : ....

Date	Client, Patient Address / ID / Serial #	Unique Botte #	Reason Notes	Admin / Dispensed By	Amount of / Waste / Hub Loss	Amount Added	Amount Used	Ending Balance
			☐ Beginning Balance Or	☐ Balance From Previous Page			↑	

VETERINARY CONTROLLED SUBSTANCE LOG

CONTROLLED SUBSTANCE : ....   STRENGTH : ....   FORM : ....

Date	Client, Patient	Address / ID / Serial #	Unique Botte #	Reason Notes	Admin / Dispensed By	Amount of / Waste / Hub Loss	Amount Added	Amount Used	Ending Balance
					☐ Beginning Balance Or	☐ Balance From Previous Page		↑	

VETERINARY CONTROLLED SUBSTANCE LOG

CONTROLLED SUBSTANCE : ....   STRENGTH : ....   FORM : ....

Date	Client, Patient	Address / ID / Serial #	Unique Botte #	Reason Notes	Admin / Dispensed By	Amount of / Waste / Hub Loss	Amount Added	Amount Used	Ending Balance
				☐ Beginning Balance Or ☐ Balance From Previous Page ⇧					

VETERINARY CONTROLLED SUBSTANCE LOG

CONTROLLED SUBSTANCE : .... STRENGTH : .... FORM : ....

Date	Client, Patient	Address / ID / Serial #	Unique Botte #	Reason Notes	Admin / Dispensed By	Amount of / Waste / Hub Loss	Amount Added	Amount Used	Ending Balance
					☐ Beginning Balance Or ☐ Balance From Previous Page ⬆				

VETERINARY CONTROLLED SUBSTANCE LOG

CONTROLLED SUBSTANCE : ....   STRENGTH : ....   FORM : ....

Date	Client, Patient	Address / ID / Serial #	Unique Botte #	Reason Notes	Admin / Dispensed By	Amount of / Waste / Hub Loss	Amount Added	Amount Used	Ending Balance
					☐ Beginning Balance Or ☐ Balance From Previous Page ⇧				

VETERINARY CONTROLLED SUBSTANCE LOG

CONTROLLED SUBSTANCE : ....   STRENGTH : ....   FORM : ....

Date	Client, Patient	Address / ID / Serial #	Unique Botte #	Reason Notes	Admin / Dispensed By	Amount of / Waste / Hub Loss	Amount Added	Amount Used	Ending Balance
					☐ Beginning Balance Or ☐ Balance From Previous Page →				

VETERINARY CONTROLLED SUBSTANCE LOG

CONTROLLED SUBSTANCE : .... STRENGTH : .... FORM : ....

Date	Client, Patient	Address / ID / Serial #	Unique Botte #	Reason Notes	Admin / Dispensed By	Amount of / Waste / Hub Loss	Amount Added	Amount Used	Ending Balance
					☐ Beginning Balance Or	☐ Balance From Previous Page ⇧			

VETERINARY CONTROLLED SUBSTANCE LOG

CONTROLLED SUBSTANCE : ....   STRENGTH : ....   FORM : ....

Date	Client, Patient	Address / ID / Serial #	Unique Bottle #	Reason Notes	Admin / Dispensed By	Amount of / Waste / Hub Loss	Amount Added	Amount Used	Ending Balance
			☐ Beginning Balance Or ☐ Balance From Previous Page ⇧						

VETERINARY CONTROLLED SUBSTANCE LOG

CONTROLLED SUBSTANCE : ....   STRENGTH : ....   FORM : ....

Date	Client, Patient	Address / ID / Serial #	Unique Botte #	Reason Notes	Admin / Dispensed By	Amount of / Waste / Hub Loss	Amount Added	Amount Used	Ending Balance
					☐ Beginning Balance Or	☐ Balance From Previous Page ⬆			

VETERINARY CONTROLLED SUBSTANCE LOG

CONTROLLED SUBSTANCE : .... STRENGTH : .... FORM : ....

Date	Client, Patient	Address / ID / Serial #	Unique Botte #	Reason Notes	Admin / Dispensed By	Amount of / Waste / Hub Loss	Amount Added	Amount Used	Ending Balance
					☐ Beginning Balance Or ☐ Balance From Previous Page				

VETERINARY CONTROLLED SUBSTANCE LOG

CONTROLLED SUBSTANCE : ....   STRENGTH : ....   FORM : ....

Date	Client, Patient	Address / ID / Serial #	Unique Botte #	Reason Notes	Admin / Dispensed By	Amount of / Waste / Hub Loss	Amount Added	Amount Used	Ending Balance
				☐ Beginning Balance Or ☐ Balance From Previous Page ⬆					

VETERINARY CONTROLLED SUBSTANCE LOG

CONTROLLED SUBSTANCE : ....   STRENGTH : ....   FORM : ....

Date	Client, Patient	Address / ID / Serial #	Unique Botte #	Reason Notes	Admin / Dispensed By	Amount of / Waste / Hub Loss	Amount Added	Amount Used	Ending Balance
				☐ Beginning Balance Or	☐ Balance From Previous Page			⇧	

VETERINARY CONTROLLED SUBSTANCE LOG

CONTROLLED SUBSTANCE : .... STRENGTH : .... FORM : ....

Date	Client, Patient	Address / ID / Serial #	Unique Botte #	Reason Notes	Admin / Dispensed By	Amount of / Waste / Hub Loss	Amount Added	Amount Used	Ending Balance
					☐ Beginning Balance Or	☐ Balance From Previous Page		⬆	

VETERINARY CONTROLLED SUBSTANCE LOG

CONTROLLED SUBSTANCE : ....   STRENGTH : ....   FORM : ....

Date	Client, Patient	Address / ID / Serial #	Unique Botte #	Reason Notes	Admin / Dispensed By	Amount of / Waste / Hub Loss	Amount Added	Amount Used	Ending Balance
					☐ Beginning Balance Or ☐ Balance From Previous Page ⬆				

VETERINARY CONTROLLED SUBSTANCE LOG

CONTROLLED SUBSTANCE : .... STRENGTH : .... FORM : ....

Date	Client, Patient	Address / ID / Serial #	Unique Botte #	Reason Notes	Admin / Dispensed By	Amount of / Waste / Hub Loss	Amount Added	Amount Used	Ending Balance
				☐ Beginning Balance Or ☐ Balance From Previous Page ⬆					

VETERINARY CONTROLLED SUBSTANCE LOG

CONTROLLED SUBSTANCE : .... STRENGTH : .... FORM : ....

Date	Client, Patient	Address / ID / Serial #	Unique Bottle #	Reason Notes	Admin / Dispensed By	Amount of / Waste / Hub Loss	Amount Added	Amount Used	Ending Balance
					☐ Beginning Balance Or ☐ Balance From Previous Page			⬆	

VETERINARY CONTROLLED SUBSTANCE LOG

CONTROLLED SUBSTANCE : ....   STRENGTH : ....   FORM : ....

Date	Client, Patient	Address / ID / Serial #	Unique Botte #	Reason Notes	Admin / Dispensed By	Amount of / Waste / Hub Loss	Amount Added	Amount Used	Ending Balance
					☐ Beginning Balance Or ☐ Balance From Previous Page ⇧				

VETERINARY CONTROLLED SUBSTANCE LOG

CONTROLLED SUBSTANCE : ....   STRENGTH : ....   FORM : ....

Date	Client, Patient	Address / ID / Serial #	Unique Botte #	Reason Notes	Admin / Dispensed By	Amount of / Waste / Hub Loss	Amount Added	Amount Used	Ending Balance
					☐ Beginning Balance Or ☐ Balance From Previous Page				

VETERINARY CONTROLLED SUBSTANCE LOG

CONTROLLED SUBSTANCE : ....   STRENGTH : ....   FORM : ....

Date	Client, Patient	Address / ID / Serial #	Unique Botte #	Reason Notes	Admin / Dispensed By	Amount of / Waste / Hub Loss	Amount Added	Amount Used	Ending Balance
				☐ Beginning Balance Or	☐ Balance From Previous Page			⇧	

VETERINARY CONTROLLED SUBSTANCE LOG

CONTROLLED SUBSTANCE : ....   STRENGTH : ....   FORM : ....

Date	Client, Patient Address / ID / Serial #	Unique Botte #	Reason Notes	Admin / Dispensed By	Amount of / Waste / Hub Loss	Amount Added	Amount Used	Ending Balance
				☐ Beginning Balance Or ☐ Balance From Previous Page ⇧				

VETERINARY CONTROLLED SUBSTANCE LOG

CONTROLLED SUBSTANCE : .... STRENGTH : .... FORM : ....

Date	Client, Patient	Address / ID / Serial #	Unique Botte #	Reason Notes	Admin / Dispensed By	Amount of / Waste / Hub Loss	Amount Added	Amount Used	Ending Balance
					☐ Beginning Balance Or ☐ Balance From Previous Page →				

VETERINARY CONTROLLED SUBSTANCE LOG

CONTROLLED SUBSTANCE : .... STRENGTH : .... FORM : ....

Date	Client, Patient Address / ID / Serial #	Unique Botte #	Reason Notes	Admin / Dispensed By	Amount of / Waste / Hub Loss	Amount Added	Amount Used	Ending Balance
				☐ Beginning Balance Or ☐ Balance From Previous Page				

VETERINARY CONTROLLED SUBSTANCE LOG

CONTROLLED SUBSTANCE : ....   STRENGTH : ....   FORM : ....

Date	Client, Patient	Address / ID / Serial #	Unique Botte #	Reason Notes	Admin / Dispensed By	Amount of / Waste / Hub Loss	Amount Added	Amount Used	Ending Balance
					☐ Beginning Balance Or ☐ Balance From Previous Page ⬆				

VETERINARY CONTROLLED SUBSTANCE LOG

CONTROLLED SUBSTANCE : ....   STRENGTH : ....   FORM : ....

Date	Client, Patient	Address / ID / Serial #	Unique Botte #	Reason Notes	Admin / Dispensed By	Amount of / Waste / Hub Loss	Amount Added	Amount Used	Ending Balance
				☐ Beginning Balance Or ☐ Balance From Previous Page ⇧					

VETERINARY CONTROLLED SUBSTANCE LOG

CONTROLLED SUBSTANCE : ....   STRENGTH : ....   FORM : ....

Date	Client, Patient	Address / ID / Serial #	Unique Botte #	Reason Notes	Admin / Dispensed By	Amount of / Waste / Hub Loss	Amount Added	Amount Used	Ending Balance
					☐ Beginning Balance Or	☐ Balance From Previous Page		⇧	

VETERINARY CONTROLLED SUBSTANCE LOG

CONTROLLED SUBSTANCE : ....   STRENGTH : ....   FORM : ....

Date	Client, Patient	Address / ID / Serial #	Unique Botte #	Reason Notes	Admin / Dispensed By	Amount of / Waste / Hub Loss	Amount Added	Amount Used	Ending Balance
					☐ Beginning Balance Or ☐ Balance From Previous Page ⇧				

VETERINARY CONTROLLED SUBSTANCE LOG

CONTROLLED SUBSTANCE : .... STRENGTH : .... FORM : ....

Date	Client, Patient	Address / ID / Serial #	Unique Botte #	Reason Notes	Admin / Dispensed By	Amount of / Waste / Hub Loss	Amount Added	Amount Used	Ending Balance
				☐ Beginning Balance Or ☐ Balance From Previous Page ⬆					

VETERINARY CONTROLLED SUBSTANCE LOG

CONTROLLED SUBSTANCE : .... STRENGTH : .... FORM : ....

Date	Client, Patient	Address / ID / Serial #	Unique Botte #	Reason Notes	Admin / Dispensed By	Amount of / Waste / Hub Loss	Amount Added	Amount Used	Ending Balance
					☐ Beginning Balance Or ☐ Balance From Previous Page ⇧				

VETERINARY CONTROLLED SUBSTANCE LOG

CONTROLLED SUBSTANCE : ....   STRENGTH : ....   FORM : ....

Date	Client, Patient	Address / ID / Serial #	Unique Botte #	Reason Notes	Admin / Dispensed By	Amount of / Waste / Hub Loss	Amount Added	Amount Used	Ending Balance
					☐ Beginning Balance Or ☐ Balance From Previous Page			⬆	

VETERINARY CONTROLLED SUBSTANCE LOG

CONTROLLED SUBSTANCE : .... STRENGTH : .... FORM : ....

Date	Client, Patient	Address / ID / Serial #	Unique Bottle #	Reason Notes	Admin / Dispensed By	Amount of / Waste / Hub Loss	Amount Added	Amount Used	Ending Balance
				☐ Beginning Balance Or	☐ Balance From Previous Page ⬆				

VETERINARY CONTROLLED SUBSTANCE LOG

CONTROLLED SUBSTANCE : ....   STRENGTH : ....   FORM : ....

Date	Client, Patient	Address / ID / Serial #	Unique Botte #	Reason Notes	Admin / Dispensed By	Amount of / Waste / Hub Loss	Amount Added	Amount Used	Ending Balance
					☐ Beginning Balance Or ☐ Balance From Previous Page ⇧				

VETERINARY CONTROLLED SUBSTANCE LOG

CONTROLLED SUBSTANCE : ....   STRENGTH : ....   FORM : ....

Date	Client, Patient	Address / ID / Serial #	Unique Botte #	Reason Notes	Admin / Dispensed By	Amount of / Waste / Hub Loss	Amount Added	Amount Used	Ending Balance
				☐ Beginning Balance Or ☐ Balance From Previous Page ⇧					

VETERINARY CONTROLLED SUBSTANCE LOG

CONTROLLED SUBSTANCE : ....   STRENGTH : ....   FORM : ....

Date	Client, Patient	Address / ID / Serial #	Unique Botte #	Reason Notes	Admin / Dispensed By	Amount of / Waste / Hub Loss	Amount Added	Amount Used	Ending Balance
					☐ Beginning Balance Or ☐ Balance From Previous Page ⇧				

VETERINARY CONTROLLED SUBSTANCE LOG

CONTROLLED SUBSTANCE : ....   STRENGTH : ....   FORM : ....

Date	Client, Patient	Address / ID / Serial #	Unique Botte #	Reason Notes	Admin / Dispensed By	Amount of / Waste / Hub Loss	Amount Added	Amount Used	Ending Balance
				☐ Beginning Balance Or ☐ Balance From Previous Page ⇧					

VETERINARY CONTROLLED SUBSTANCE LOG

CONTROLLED SUBSTANCE : .... STRENGTH : .... FORM : ....

Date	Client, Patient	Address / ID / Serial #	Unique Botte #	Reason Notes	Admin / Dispensed By	Amount of / Waste / Hub Loss	Amount Added	Amount Used	Ending Balance
					☐ Beginning Balance Or ☐ Balance From Previous Page ⬆				

VETERINARY CONTROLLED SUBSTANCE LOG

CONTROLLED SUBSTANCE : ....   STRENGTH : ....   FORM : ....

Date	Client, Patient	Address / ID / Serial #	Unique Botte #	Reason Notes	Admin / Dispensed By	Amount of / Waste / Hub Loss	Amount Added	Amount Used	Ending Balance
				☐ Beginning Balance Or ☐ Balance From Previous Page					

VETERINARY CONTROLLED SUBSTANCE LOG

CONTROLLED SUBSTANCE : ....   STRENGTH : ....   FORM : ....

Date	Client, Patient	Address / ID / Serial #	Unique Botte #	Reason Notes	Admin / Dispensed By	Amount of / Waste / Hub Loss	Amount Added	Amount Used	Ending Balance
					☐ Beginning Balance Or ☐ Balance From Previous Page ⇧				

VETERINARY CONTROLLED SUBSTANCE LOG

CONTROLLED SUBSTANCE : ....   STRENGTH : ....   FORM : ....

Date	Client, Patient	Address / ID / Serial #	Unique Botte #	Reason Notes	Admin / Dispensed By	Amount of / Waste / Hub Loss	Amount Added	Amount Used	Ending Balance
					☐ Beginning Balance Or ☐ Balance From Previous Page ⬆				

VETERINARY CONTROLLED SUBSTANCE LOG

CONTROLLED SUBSTANCE : ....   STRENGTH : ....   FORM : ....

Date	Client, Patient	Address / ID / Serial #	Unique Botte #	Reason Notes	Admin / Dispensed By	Amount of / Waste / Hub Loss	Amount Added	Amount Used	Ending Balance
					☐ Beginning Balance Or	☐ Balance From Previous Page		⇧	

VETERINARY CONTROLLED SUBSTANCE LOG

CONTROLLED SUBSTANCE : ....   STRENGTH : ....   FORM : ....

Date	Client, Patient	Address / ID / Serial #	Unique Botte #	Reason Notes	Admin / Dispensed By	Amount of / Waste / Hub Loss	Amount Added	Amount Used	Ending Balance
					☐ Beginning Balance Or ☐ Balance From Previous Page				

VETERINARY CONTROLLED SUBSTANCE LOG

CONTROLLED SUBSTANCE : .... STRENGTH : .... FORM : ....

Date	Client, Patient Address / ID / Serial #	Unique Botte #	Reason Notes	Admin / Dispensed By	Amount of / Waste / Hub Loss	Amount Added	Amount Used	Ending Balance
			☐ Beginning Balance Or ☐ Balance From Previous Page ⇧					

VETERINARY CONTROLLED SUBSTANCE LOG

CONTROLLED SUBSTANCE : .... STRENGTH : .... FORM : ....

Date	Client, Patient	Address / ID / Serial #	Unique Botte #	Reason Notes	Admin / Dispensed By	Amount of / Waste / Hub Loss	Amount Added	Amount Used	Ending Balance
					☐ Beginning Balance Or ☐ Balance From Previous Page ⇦				

VETERINARY CONTROLLED SUBSTANCE LOG

CONTROLLED SUBSTANCE : .... STRENGTH : .... FORM : ....

Date	Client, Patient	Address / ID / Serial #	Unique Botte #	Reason Notes	Admin / Dispensed By	Amount of / Waste / Hub Loss	Amount Added	Amount Used	Ending Balance
					☐ Beginning Balance Or ☐ Balance From Previous Page				

VETERINARY CONTROLLED SUBSTANCE LOG

CONTROLLED SUBSTANCE : ....   STRENGTH : ....   FORM : ....

Date	Client, Patient	Address / ID / Serial #	Unique Botte #	Reason Notes	Admin / Dispensed By	Amount of / Waste / Hub Loss	Amount Added	Amount Used	Ending Balance
					☐ Beginning Balance Or	☐ Balance From Previous Page		⬆	

VETERINARY CONTROLLED SUBSTANCE LOG

CONTROLLED SUBSTANCE : ....   STRENGTH : ....   FORM : ....

Date	Client, Patient	Address / ID / Serial #	Unique Botte #	Reason Notes	Admin / Dispensed By	Amount of / Waste / Hub Loss	Amount Added	Amount Used	Ending Balance
					☐ Beginning Balance Or ☐ Balance From Previous Page			⇧	

VETERINARY CONTROLLED SUBSTANCE LOG

CONTROLLED SUBSTANCE : ....   STRENGTH : ....   FORM : ....

Date	Client, Patient Address / ID / Serial #	Unique Botte #	Reason Notes	Admin / Dispensed By	Amount of / Waste / Hub Loss	Amount Added	Amount Used	Ending Balance
				☐ Beginning Balance Or ☐ Balance From Previous Page ⇧				

VETERINARY CONTROLLED SUBSTANCE LOG

CONTROLLED SUBSTANCE : .... STRENGTH : .... FORM : ....

Date	Client, Patient	Address / ID / Serial #	Unique Botte #	Reason Notes	Admin / Dispensed By	Amount of / Waste / Hub Loss	Amount Added	Amount Used	Ending Balance
					☐ Beginning Balance Or ☐ Balance From Previous Page				

VETERINARY CONTROLLED SUBSTANCE LOG

CONTROLLED SUBSTANCE : .... STRENGTH : .... FORM : ....

Date	Client, Patient	Address / ID / Serial #	Unique Botte #	Reason Notes	Admin / Dispensed By	Amount of / Waste / Hub Loss	Amount Added	Amount Used	Ending Balance
					☐ Beginning Balance Or	☐ Balance From Previous Page		⇧	

VETERINARY CONTROLLED SUBSTANCE LOG

CONTROLLED SUBSTANCE : .... STRENGTH : .... FORM : ....

Date	Client, Patient	Address / ID / Serial #	Unique Botte #	Reason Notes	Admin / Dispensed By	Amount of / Waste / Hub Loss	Amount Added	Amount Used	Ending Balance
					☐ Beginning Balance Or ☐ Balance From Previous Page ⬆				

VETERINARY CONTROLLED SUBSTANCE LOG

CONTROLLED SUBSTANCE : .... STRENGTH : .... FORM : ....

Date	Client, Patient	Address / ID / Serial #	Unique Botte #	Reason Notes	Admin / Dispensed By	Amount of / Waste / Hub Loss	Amount Added	Amount Used	Ending Balance
					☐ Beginning Balance Or ☐ Balance From Previous Page ⬆				

VETERINARY CONTROLLED SUBSTANCE LOG

CONTROLLED SUBSTANCE : ....   STRENGTH : ....   FORM : ....

Date	Client, Patient	Address / ID / Serial #	Unique Botte #	Reason Notes	Admin / Dispensed By	Amount of / Waste / Hub Loss	Amount Added	Amount Used	Ending Balance
					☐ Beginning Balance Or ☐ Balance From Previous Page ⬆				

VETERINARY CONTROLLED SUBSTANCE LOG

CONTROLLED SUBSTANCE : .... STRENGTH : .... FORM : ....

Date	Client, Patient	Address / ID / Serial #	Unique Botte #	Reason Notes	Admin / Dispensed By	Amount of / Waste / Hub Loss	Amount Added	Amount Used	Ending Balance
			☐ Beginning Balance Or		☐ Balance From Previous Page	⇧			

VETERINARY CONTROLLED SUBSTANCE LOG

CONTROLLED SUBSTANCE : ....   STRENGTH : ....   FORM : ....

Date	Client, Patient	Address / ID / Serial #	Unique Botte #	Reason Notes	Admin / Dispensed By	Amount of / Waste / Hub Loss	Amount Added	Amount Used	Ending Balance
					☐ Beginning Balance Or ☐ Balance From Previous Page →				

VETERINARY CONTROLLED SUBSTANCE LOG

CONTROLLED SUBSTANCE : ....   STRENGTH : ....   FORM : ....

Date	Client, Patient	Address / ID / Serial #	Unique Botte #	Reason Notes	Admin / Dispensed By	Amount of / Waste / Hub Loss	Amount Added	Amount Used	Ending Balance
					☐ Beginning Balance Or ☐ Balance From Previous Page			⇧	

VETERINARY CONTROLLED SUBSTANCE LOG

CONTROLLED SUBSTANCE : ....

STRENGTH : ....

FORM : ....

Date	Client, Patient	Address / ID / Serial #	Unique Botte #	Reason Notes	Admin / Dispensed By	Amount of / Waste / Hub Loss	Amount Added	Amount Used	Ending Balance
					☐ Beginning Balance Or ☐ Balance From Previous Page ⬆				

VETERINARY CONTROLLED SUBSTANCE LOG

CONTROLLED SUBSTANCE : ....   STRENGTH : ....   FORM : ....

Date	Client, Patient	Address / ID / Serial #	Unique Botte #	Reason Notes	Admin / Dispensed By	Amount of / Waste / Hub Loss	Amount Added	Amount Used	Ending Balance
					☐ Beginning Balance Or ☐ Balance From Previous Page ⇧				

Veterinary Controlled Substance Log

CONTROLLED SUBSTANCE : .... STRENGTH : .... FORM : ....

Date	Client, Patient Address / ID / Serial #	Unique Botte #	Reason Notes	Admin / Dispensed By	Amount of / Waste / Hub Loss	Amount Added	Amount Used	Ending Balance
				☐ Beginning Balance Or	☐ Balance From Previous Page ⬆			

VETERINARY CONTROLLED SUBSTANCE LOG

CONTROLLED SUBSTANCE : .... STRENGTH : .... FORM : ....

Date	Client, Patient	Address / ID / Serial #	Unique Bottle #	Reason Notes	Admin / Dispensed By	Amount of / Waste / Hub Loss	Amount Added	Amount Used	Ending Balance
					☐ Beginning Balance Or ☐ Balance From Previous Page ⇧				

VETERINARY CONTROLLED SUBSTANCE LOG

CONTROLLED SUBSTANCE : ....   STRENGTH : ....   FORM : ....

Date	Client, Patient	Address / ID / Serial #	Unique Botte #	Reason Notes	Admin / Dispensed By	Amount of / Waste / Hub Loss	Amount Added	Amount Used	Ending Balance
					☐ Beginning Balance Or	☐ Balance From Previous Page ⇧			

VETERINARY CONTROLLED SUBSTANCE LOG

CONTROLLED SUBSTANCE : .... STRENGTH : .... FORM : ....

Date	Client, Patient	Address / ID / Serial #	Unique Botte #	Reason Notes	Admin / Dispensed By	Amount of / Waste / Hub Loss	Amount Added	Amount Used	Ending Balance
					☐ Beginning Balance Or	☐ Balance From Previous Page			

VETERINARY CONTROLLED SUBSTANCE LOG

CONTROLLED SUBSTANCE : .... STRENGTH : .... FORM : ....

Date	Client, Patient	Address / ID / Serial #	Unique Botte #	Reason Notes	Admin / Dispensed By	Amount of / Waste / Hub Loss	Amount Added	Amount Used	Ending Balance
					☐ Beginning Balance Or ☐ Balance From Previous Page ⇧				

VETERINARY CONTROLLED SUBSTANCE LOG

CONTROLLED SUBSTANCE : .... STRENGTH : .... FORM : ....

Date	Client, Patient	Address / ID / Serial #	Unique Botte #	Reason Notes	Admin / Dispensed By	Amount of / Waste / Hub Loss	Amount Added	Amount Used	Ending Balance
					☐ Beginning Balance Or ☐ Balance From Previous Page ⬆				

VETERINARY CONTROLLED SUBSTANCE LOG

CONTROLLED SUBSTANCE : ....   STRENGTH : ....   FORM : ....

Date	Client, Patient	Address / ID / Serial #	Unique Botte #	Reason Notes	Admin / Dispensed By	Amount of / Waste / Hub Loss	Amount Added	Amount Used	Ending Balance
					☐ Beginning Balance Or ☐ Balance From Previous Page ⬆				

VETERINARY CONTROLLED SUBSTANCE LOG

CONTROLLED SUBSTANCE : .... STRENGTH : .... FORM : ....

Date	Client, Patient	Address / ID / Serial #	Unique Botte #	Reason Notes	Admin / Dispensed By	Amount of / Waste / Hub Loss	Amount Added	Amount Used	Ending Balance
					☐ Beginning Balance Or ☐ Balance From Previous Page ⇧				

VETERINARY CONTROLLED SUBSTANCE LOG

CONTROLLED SUBSTANCE : ....   STRENGTH : ....   FORM : ....

Date	Client, Patient	Address / ID / Serial #	Unique Botte #	Reason Notes	Admin / Dispensed By	Amount of / Waste / Hub Loss	Amount Added	Amount Used	Ending Balance
					☐ Beginning Balance Or ☐ Balance From Previous Page			⬆	

VETERINARY CONTROLLED SUBSTANCE LOG

CONTROLLED SUBSTANCE : .... STRENGTH : .... FORM : ....

Date	Client, Patient	Address / ID / Serial #	Unique Botte #	Reason Notes	Admin / Dispensed By	Amount of / Waste / Hub Loss	Amount Added	Amount Used	Ending Balance
					☐ Beginning Balance Or ☐ Balance From Previous Page ⬆				

VETERINARY CONTROLLED SUBSTANCE LOG

CONTROLLED SUBSTANCE : ....   STRENGTH : ....   FORM : ....

Date	Client, Patient	Address / ID / Serial #	Unique Botte #	Reason Notes	Admin / Dispensed By	Amount of / Waste / Hub Loss	Amount Added	Amount Used	Ending Balance
					☐ Beginning Balance Or ☐ Balance From Previous Page ⇦				

VETERINARY CONTROLLED SUBSTANCE LOG

CONTROLLED SUBSTANCE : ....   STRENGTH : ....   FORM : ....

Date	Client, Patient	Address / ID / Serial #	Unique Botte #	Reason Notes	Admin / Dispensed By	Amount of / Waste / Hub Loss	Amount Added	Amount Used	Ending Balance
					☐ Beginning Balance Or ☐ Balance From Previous Page			⇧	

VETERINARY CONTROLLED SUBSTANCE LOG

CONTROLLED SUBSTANCE : .... STRENGTH : .... FORM : ....

Date	Client, Patient	Address / ID / Serial #	Unique Botte #	Reason Notes	Admin / Dispensed By	Amount of / Waste / Hub Loss	Amount Added	Amount Used	Ending Balance
					☐ Beginning Balance Or ☐ Balance From Previous Page ⬆				

VETERINARY CONTROLLED SUBSTANCE LOG

CONTROLLED SUBSTANCE : .... STRENGTH : .... FORM : ....

Date	Client, Patient	Address / ID / Serial #	Unique Botte #	Reason Notes	Admin / Dispensed By	Amount of / Waste / Hub Loss	Amount Added	Amount Used	Ending Balance
				☐ Beginning Balance Or ☐ Balance From Previous Page ⇧					

VETERINARY CONTROLLED SUBSTANCE LOG

CONTROLLED SUBSTANCE : ....

STRENGTH : ....

FORM : ....

Date	Client, Patient	Address / ID / Serial #	Unique Botte #	Reason Notes	Admin / Dispensed By	Amount of / Waste / Hub Loss	Amount Added	Amount Used	Ending Balance
					☐ Beginning Balance Or ☐ Balance From Previous Page →				

VETERINARY CONTROLLED SUBSTANCE LOG

CONTROLLED SUBSTANCE : ....   STRENGTH : ....   FORM : ....

Date	Client, Patient	Address / ID / Serial #	Unique Botte #	Reason Notes	Admin / Dispensed By	Amount of / Waste / Hub Loss	Amount Added	Amount Used	Ending Balance
					☐ Beginning Balance Or ☐ Balance From Previous Page ⇧				

VETERINARY CONTROLLED SUBSTANCE LOG

CONTROLLED SUBSTANCE : ....

STRENGTH : ....

FORM : ....

Date	Client, Patient	Address / ID / Serial #	Unique Botte #	Reason Notes	Admin / Dispensed By	Amount of / Waste / Hub Loss	Amount Added	Amount Used	Ending Balance
					☐ Beginning Balance Or ☐ Balance From Previous Page ⇧				

VETERINARY CONTROLLED SUBSTANCE LOG

CONTROLLED SUBSTANCE : .... STRENGTH : .... FORM : ....

Date	Client, Patient	Address / ID / Serial #	Unique Botte #	Reason Notes	Admin / Dispensed By	Amount of / Waste / Hub Loss	Amount Added	Amount Used	Ending Balance
				☐ Beginning Balance Or ☐ Balance From Previous Page ⇧					

VETERINARY CONTROLLED SUBSTANCE LOG

CONTROLLED SUBSTANCE : .... STRENGTH : .... FORM : ....

Date	Client, Patient	Address / ID / Serial #	Unique Botte #	Reason Notes	Admin / Dispensed By	Amount of / Waste / Hub Loss	Amount Added	Amount Used	Ending Balance
				☐ Beginning Balance Or ☐ Balance From Previous Page ⬆					

VETERINARY CONTROLLED SUBSTANCE LOG

CONTROLLED SUBSTANCE : .... STRENGTH : .... FORM : ....

Date	Client, Patient	Address / ID / Serial #	Unique Botte #	Reason Notes	Admin / Dispensed By	Amount of / Waste / Hub Loss	Amount Added	Amount Used	Ending Balance
				☐ Beginning Balance Or	☐ Balance From Previous Page			⬆	

VETERINARY CONTROLLED SUBSTANCE LOG

CONTROLLED SUBSTANCE : .... STRENGTH : .... FORM : ....

Date	Client, Patient	Address / ID / Serial #	Unique Botte #	Reason Notes	Admin / Dispensed By	Amount of / Waste / Hub Loss	Amount Added	Amount Used	Ending Balance
					☐ Beginning Balance Or ☐ Balance From Previous Page ⇧				

VETERINARY CONTROLLED SUBSTANCE LOG

CONTROLLED SUBSTANCE : ....   STRENGTH : ....   FORM : ....

Date	Client, Patient	Address / ID / Serial #	Unique Botte #	Reason Notes	Admin / Dispensed By	Amount of / Waste / Hub Loss	Amount Added	Amount Used	Ending Balance
					☐ Beginning Balance Or ☐ Balance From Previous Page ⇧				

VETERINARY CONTROLLED SUBSTANCE LOG

CONTROLLED SUBSTANCE : ....   STRENGTH : ....   FORM : ....

Date	Client, Patient	Address / ID / Serial #	Unique Botte #	Reason Notes	Admin / Dispensed By	Amount of / Waste / Hub Loss	Amount Added	Amount Used	Ending Balance
				☐ Beginning Balance Or ☐ Balance From Previous Page ⇧					

Veterinary Controlled Substance Log

CONTROLLED SUBSTANCE : ....   STRENGTH : ....   FORM : ....

Date	Client, Patient	Address / ID / Serial #	Unique Botte #	Reason Notes	Admin / Dispensed By	Amount of / Waste / Hub Loss	Amount Added	Amount Used	Ending Balance
			☐ Beginning Balance Or	☐ Balance From Previous Page				⇧	

VETERINARY CONTROLLED SUBSTANCE LOG

CONTROLLED SUBSTANCE : ....   STRENGTH : ....   FORM : ....

Date	Client, Patient	Address / ID / Serial #	Unique Botte #	Reason Notes	Admin / Dispensed By	Amount of / Waste / Hub Loss	Amount Added	Amount Used	Ending Balance
				☐ Beginning Balance Or ☐ Balance From Previous Page ⇧					

VETERINARY CONTROLLED SUBSTANCE LOG

CONTROLLED SUBSTANCE : .... STRENGTH : .... FORM : ....

Date	Client, Patient	Address / ID / Serial #	Unique Botte #	Reason Notes	Admin / Dispensed By	Amount of / Waste / Hub Loss	Amount Added	Amount Used	Ending Balance
					☐ Beginning Balance Or ☐ Balance From Previous Page ⇧				

VETERINARY CONTROLLED SUBSTANCE LOG

CONTROLLED SUBSTANCE : .... STRENGTH : .... FORM : ....

Date	Client, Patient	Address / ID / Serial #	Unique Botte #	Reason Notes	Admin / Dispensed By	Amount of / Waste / Hub Loss	Amount Added	Amount Used	Ending Balance
					☐ Beginning Balance Or ☐ Balance From Previous Page ⇧				

VETERINARY CONTROLLED SUBSTANCE LOG

CONTROLLED SUBSTANCE : .... STRENGTH : .... FORM : ....

Date	Client, Patient	Address / ID / Serial #	Unique Botte #	Reason Notes	Admin / Dispensed By	Amount of / Waste / Hub Loss	Amount Added	Amount Used	Ending Balance
				☐ Beginning Balance Or ☐ Balance From Previous Page ⇧					

VETERINARY CONTROLLED SUBSTANCE LOG

CONTROLLED SUBSTANCE : .... STRENGTH : .... FORM : ....

Date	Client, Patient	Address / ID / Serial #	Unique Botte #	Reason Notes	Admin / Dispensed By	Amount of / Waste / Hub Loss	Amount Added	Amount Used	Ending Balance
					☐ Beginning Balance Or	☐ Balance From Previous Page			

VETERINARY CONTROLLED SUBSTANCE LOG

CONTROLLED SUBSTANCE : .... STRENGTH : .... FORM : ....

Date	Client, Patient	Address / ID / Serial #	Unique Botte #	Reason Notes	Admin / Dispensed By	Amount of / Waste / Hub Loss	Amount Added	Amount Used	Ending Balance
			☐ Beginning Balance Or	☐ Balance From Previous Page	⬆				

VETERINARY CONTROLLED SUBSTANCE LOG

CONTROLLED SUBSTANCE : .... STRENGTH : .... FORM : ....

Date	Client, Patient	Address / ID / Serial #	Unique Botte #	Reason Notes	Admin / Dispensed By	Amount of / Waste / Hub Loss	Amount Added	Amount Used	Ending Balance
					☐ Beginning Balance Or ☐ Balance From Previous Page ⇧				

VETERINARY CONTROLLED SUBSTANCE LOG

CONTROLLED SUBSTANCE : ....   STRENGTH : ....   FORM : ....

Date	Client, Patient Address / ID / Serial #	Unique Botte #	Reason Notes	Admin / Dispensed By	Amount of / Waste / Hub Loss	Amount Added	Amount Used	Ending Balance
				☐ Beginning Balance Or ☐ Balance From Previous Page ⬆				

VETERINARY CONTROLLED SUBSTANCE LOG

CONTROLLED SUBSTANCE : .... STRENGTH : .... FORM : ....

Date	Client, Patient	Address / ID / Serial #	Unique Botte #	Reason Notes	Admin / Dispensed By	Amount of / Waste / Hub Loss	Amount Added	Amount Used	Ending Balance
					☐ Beginning Balance Or ☐ Balance From Previous Page ⇧				

VETERINARY CONTROLLED SUBSTANCE LOG

CONTROLLED SUBSTANCE : ....   STRENGTH : ....   FORM : ....

Date	Client, Patient	Address / ID / Serial #	Unique Botte #	Reason Notes	Admin / Dispensed By	Amount of / Waste / Hub Loss	Amount Added	Amount Used	Ending Balance
				☐ Beginning Balance Or ☐ Balance From Previous Page					

VETERINARY CONTROLLED SUBSTANCE LOG

CONTROLLED SUBSTANCE : ....   STRENGTH : ....   FORM : ....

Date	Client, Patient	Address / ID / Serial #	Unique Botte #	Reason Notes	Admin / Dispensed By	Amount of / Waste / Hub Loss	Amount Added	Amount Used	Ending Balance
				□ Beginning Balance Or □ Balance From Previous Page ⇦					

VETERINARY CONTROLLED SUBSTANCE LOG

CONTROLLED SUBSTANCE : .... STRENGTH : .... FORM : ....

Date	Client, Patient	Address / ID / Serial #	Unique Botte #	Reason Notes	Admin / Dispensed By	Amount of / Waste / Hub Loss	Amount Added	Amount Used	Ending Balance
					☐ Beginning Balance Or ☐ Balance From Previous Page ⇧				

VETERINARY CONTROLLED SUBSTANCE LOG

CONTROLLED SUBSTANCE : .... STRENGTH : .... FORM : ....

Date	Client, Patient	Address / ID / Serial #	Unique Botte #	Reason Notes	Admin / Dispensed By	Amount of / Waste / Hub Loss	Amount Added	Amount Used	Ending Balance
					☐ Beginning Balance Or ☐ Balance From Previous Page ⇦				

VETERINARY CONTROLLED SUBSTANCE LOG

CONTROLLED SUBSTANCE : ....   STRENGTH : ....   FORM : ....

Date	Client, Patient	Address / ID / Serial #	Unique Botte #	Reason Notes	Admin / Dispensed By	Amount of / Waste / Hub Loss	Amount Added	Amount Used	Ending Balance
				☐ Beginning Balance Or ☐ Balance From Previous Page ⇧					

VETERINARY CONTROLLED SUBSTANCE LOG

CONTROLLED SUBSTANCE : .... STRENGTH : .... FORM : ....

Date	Client, Patient Address / ID / Serial #	Unique Botte #	Reason Notes	Admin / Dispensed By	Amount of / Waste / Hub Loss	Amount Added	Amount Used	Ending Balance
				□ Beginning Balance Or □ Balance From Previous Page ⇦				

VETERINARY CONTROLLED SUBSTANCE LOG

CONTROLLED SUBSTANCE : .... STRENGTH : .... FORM : ....

Date	Client, Patient	Address / ID / Serial #	Unique Botte #	Reason Notes	Admin / Dispensed By	Amount of / Waste / Hub Loss	Amount Added	Amount Used	Ending Balance
				☐ Beginning Balance Or ☐ Balance From Previous Page ⬆					

VETERINARY CONTROLLED SUBSTANCE LOG

CONTROLLED SUBSTANCE : .... STRENGTH : .... FORM : ....

Date	Client, Patient	Address / ID / Serial #	Unique Botte #	Reason Notes	Admin / Dispensed By	Amount of / Waste / Hub Loss	Amount Added	Amount Used	Ending Balance
				☐ Beginning Balance Or ☐ Balance From Previous Page ⇧					

VETERINARY CONTROLLED SUBSTANCE LOG

CONTROLLED SUBSTANCE : .... STRENGTH : .... FORM : ....

Date	Client, Patient	Address / ID / Serial #	Unique Botte #	Reason Notes	Admin / Dispensed By	Amount of / Waste / Hub Loss	Amount Added	Amount Used	Ending Balance
					□ Beginning Balance Or	□ Balance From Previous Page ⇧			

VETERINARY CONTROLLED SUBSTANCE LOG

CONTROLLED SUBSTANCE : .... STRENGTH : .... FORM : ....

Date	Client, Patient Address / ID / Serial #	Unique Bottle #	Reason Notes	Admin / Dispensed By	Amount of / Waste / Hub Loss	Amount Added	Amount Used	Ending Balance
			☐ Beginning Balance Or ☐ Balance From Previous Page					

VETERINARY CONTROLLED SUBSTANCE LOG

CONTROLLED SUBSTANCE : .... STRENGTH : .... FORM : ....

Date	Client, Patient	Address / ID / Serial #	Unique Botte #	Reason Notes	Admin / Dispensed By	Amount of / Waste / Hub Loss	Amount Added	Amount Used	Ending Balance
				☐ Beginning Balance Or	☐ Balance From Previous Page			↑	

VETERINARY CONTROLLED SUBSTANCE LOG

CONTROLLED SUBSTANCE : ....   STRENGTH : ....   FORM : ....

Date	Client, Patient	Address / ID / Serial #	Unique Botte #	Reason Notes	Admin / Dispensed By	Amount of / Waste / Hub Loss	Amount Added	Amount Used	Ending Balance
					☐ Beginning Balance Or ☐ Balance From Previous Page ⇧				

VETERINARY CONTROLLED SUBSTANCE LOG

CONTROLLED SUBSTANCE : ....   STRENGTH : ....   FORM : ....

Date	Client, Patient	Address / ID / Serial #	Unique Botte #	Reason Notes	Admin / Dispensed By	Amount of / Waste / Hub Loss	Amount Added	Amount Used	Ending Balance
				☐ Beginning Balance Or ☐ Balance From Previous Page					

VETERINARY CONTROLLED SUBSTANCE LOG

CONTROLLED SUBSTANCE : ....   STRENGTH : ....   FORM : ....

Date	Client, Patient	Address / ID / Serial #	Unique Botte #	Reason Notes	Admin / Dispensed By	Amount of / Waste / Hub Loss	Amount Added	Amount Used	Ending Balance
					☐ Beginning Balance Or ☐ Balance From Previous Page ⇧				

Made in the USA
Las Vegas, NV
02 December 2024

13205730R00068